RICHA YADAV

Nourish Your Thyroid: A Guide to Healing through Nutrition and Lifestyle

Optimize well-being through nutrition. Lifestyle tips for a balanced thyroid and vibrant, energetic living

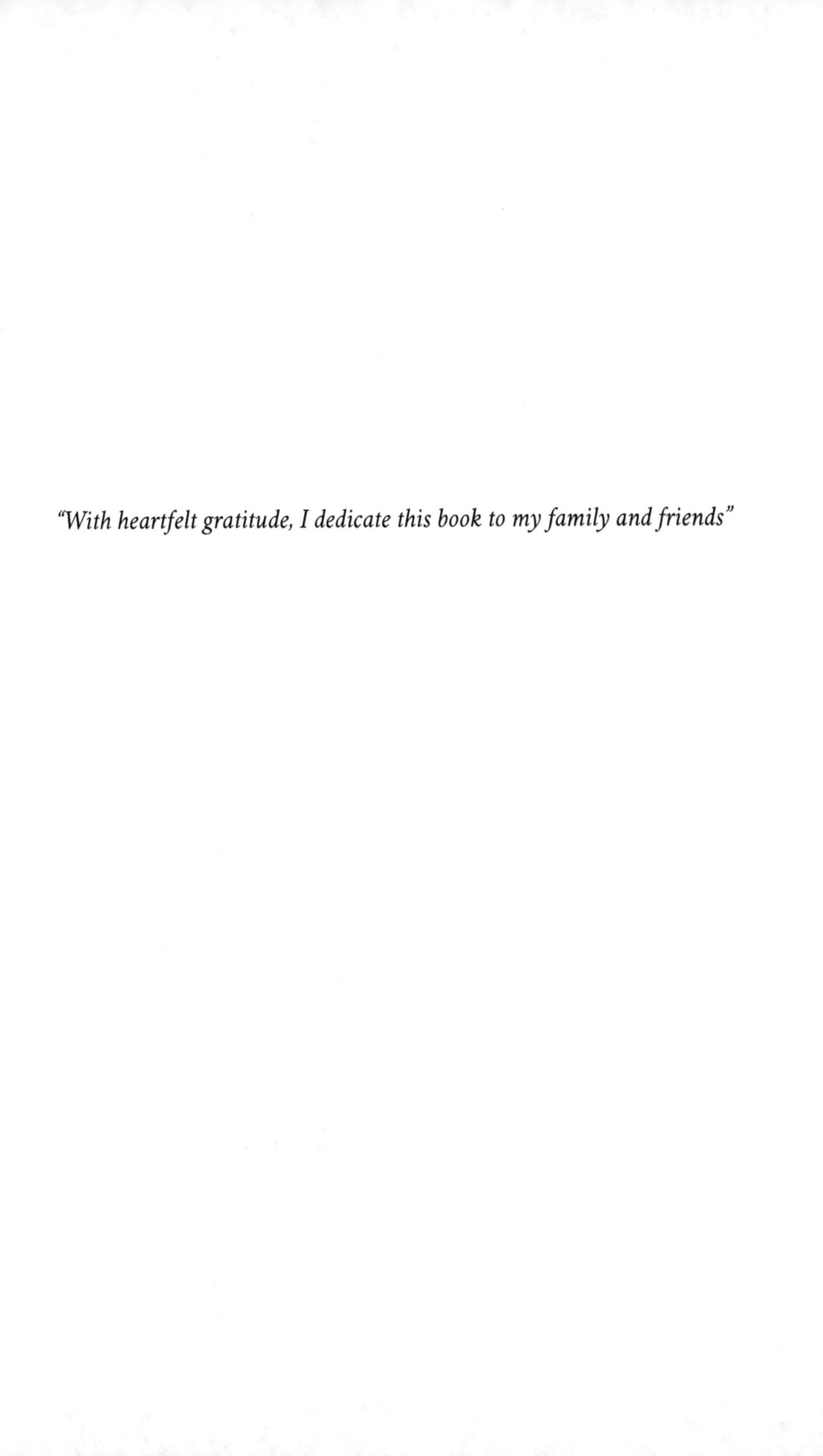

"With heartfelt gratitude, I dedicate this book to my family and friends"

"A person is said to have achieved yoga, the union with the divine, when moderation is established in eating and recreation, with balanced effort in actions, and when sleep and wakefulness are regulated. This discipline destroys suffering." - Bhagavad Gita (6.17)

Contents

Foreword

Preface

Acknowledgement

1

INTRODUCTION

In a world that often races against time, our health can become a casualty of our fast-paced lives. The thyroid, a small but mighty gland nestled in our necks, plays a pivotal role in maintaining our overall well-being. Yet, it is a frequently overlooked and misunderstood aspect of our health. Welcome to "Nourish Your Thyroid: A Guide to Healing Through Nutrition," your comprehensive journey into understanding and revitalizing one of the body's unsung heroes.

This book is not just about the thyroid; it is a roadmap to reclaiming your vitality and well-being through the power of intentional nutrition.

In the following pages, we will delve into the intricate connection between your thyroid and the food you consume. You will discover the profound impact that nutrition can have on your thyroid function, influencing everything from energy levels and metabolism to mental clarity and emotional balance. This book is not a one-size-fits-all solution; rather, it is a guide that empowers you to make informed choices, customized to your unique needs.

Whether you are facing thyroid issues or are proactively seeking to optimize your health, "Nourish Your Thyroid" is designed to be your companion in this transformative journey. I will share insights, practical tips, and delicious recipes to help you embrace a thyroid-friendly lifestyle. From understanding the role of key nutrients to crafting meals that support thyroid health, each chapter is crafted to demystify the science and make nutrition an accessible tool for your well-being.

Together, let us embark on a path of healing and nourishment. Your thyroid deserves the best, and this book is your guide to unlocking the transformative potential of nutrition on your journey to optimal health.

Several years ago, I found myself navigating the challenging terrain of thyroid dysfunction. The fatigue was relentless, my energy levels plummeted, and a fog of confusion settled over my daily life. Doctor visits became a routine, each one marked by the frustration of inconclusive diagnoses and fleeting solutions. It was during this time that I stumbled upon the transformative power of nutrition in healing the thyroid.

My journey wasn't just about adopting a new diet; it was a profound shift in perspective. As I began to explore the intricate connection between my thyroid and the foods I consumed, the pieces of the puzzle started to fall into place. Personal triumphs and setbacks alike became valuable lessons, shaping the foundation of the knowledge I now share with you in these pages.

2

Chapter 1: Understanding the Thyroid

The Thyroid Gland: A Master of Metabolism

In the intricate tapestry of our body's internal orchestra, the thyroid gland stands as a conductor, orchestrating the symphony of metabolism. Nestled discreetly in the lower front part of the neck, this butterfly-shaped gland plays a pivotal role in maintaining equilibrium within our intricate biological system.

Unveiling the Anatomy

Before we delve into its significance, let's unravel the anatomical marvel that is the thyroid gland. Composed of two lobes connected by a thin strip of tissue called the isthmus, the thyroid is intricately positioned just below the Adam's apple. Tiny in size but colossal in impact, it houses an arsenal of follicles that resemble microscopic spheres, where the magic of thyroid hormone synthesis takes place.

The Thyroid's Orchestra: Hormones at Play

At the heart of the thyroid's influence are two key hormones: thyroxine (T4) and triiodothyronine (T3). These hormones act as messengers, transmitting signals to cells throughout the body to regulate essential processes such as metabolism, energy production, and temperature control. In essence, the thyroid hormones are the conductors directing the pace at which our body's engines run.

A Balancing Act: The Hypothalamus-Pituitary-Thyroid Axis

To truly comprehend the thyroid's role, we must acknowledge the intricate dance it engages in with the hypothalamus and pituitary gland. This triumvirate forms the Hypothalamus-Pituitary-Thyroid (HPT) axis, a dynamic feedback loop that ensures the thyroid functions optimally. When the body senses a drop in thyroid hormone levels, the hypothalamus releases thyrotropin-releasing hormone (TRH), signaling the pituitary gland to produce thyroid-stimulating hormone (TSH). TSH, in turn, nudges the thyroid to increase hormone production, thereby restoring balance.

The Symphony of Metabolism

Picture the thyroid as the maestro of metabolism, fine-tuning the body's energy expenditure, cellular repair, and growth. When in harmony, the thyroid ensures our systems hum along at an optimal tempo. However, when this delicate equilibrium is disrupted, the consequences ripple through our well-being, leading to a spectrum of thyroid disorders.

Unlocking the Mysteries

As we embark on this journey to understand the thyroid, we will demystify the common disorders that can impact its function. From hypothyroidism, where the gland underperforms, to hyperthyroidism, characterized by an overactive thyroid, each condition paints a unique portrait of the thyroid's significance in our health.

In the chapters that follow, we will explore how nutrition can be a powerful ally in maintaining thyroid health. But first, let us grasp the essence of this intricate gland, decipher its language, and appreciate the symphony it orchestrates within us.

Common Thyroid Disorders

1. Hypothyroidism:
   Overview:
   Hypothyroidism refers to an underactive thyroid, where the gland fails to produce sufficient thyroid hormones, primarily thyroxine (T4) and triiodothyronine (T3).
   Causes:

- Autoimmune thyroiditis (Hashimoto's thyroiditis)
- Iodine deficiency
- Congenital hypothyroidism
- Certain medications and treatments

Symptoms:

- Fatigue
- Weight gain
- Cold intolerance
- Dry skin and hair
- Depression
- Muscle weakness

Management:
Treatment typically involves thyroid hormone replacement therapy

to supplement the insufficient production of hormones.

2. Hyperthyroidism:

Overview:

Hyperthyroidism is the opposite of hypothyroidism, characterized by an overactive thyroid gland, leading to excessive production of thyroid hormones.

Causes:

- Graves' disease (autoimmune disorder)
- Thyroid nodules
- Inflammation of the thyroid (thyroiditis)

Symptoms:

- Weight loss
- Rapid heartbeat
- Anxiety and irritability
- Tremors
- Heat intolerance
- Sweating

Management:

Treatment options may include medications to regulate hormone levels, radioactive iodine therapy, or, in severe cases, surgical removal of the thyroid gland.

3. Hashimoto's Thyroiditis:

Overview:

Hashimoto's thyroiditis is an autoimmune condition where the body's immune system mistakenly attacks the thyroid gland, leading to chronic inflammation and gradual destruction of thyroid tissue.

Causes:

- Genetic predisposition
- Environmental factors
- Imbalance in the immune system

Symptoms:

- Fatigue
- Weight gain
- Swelling of the thyroid (goiter)
- Thinning hair
- Joint and muscle pain
- Sensitivity to cold

Management:

While there is no cure for Hashimoto's, treatment often involves thyroid hormone replacement therapy to address hormone deficiencies and manage symptoms. Lifestyle and dietary changes may also play a role in managing the autoimmune response.

Understanding these common thyroid disorders lays the foundation for exploring how nutrition can be a crucial component in managing and supporting thyroid health. In the chapters ahead, we will delve into the specific dietary strategies that can positively impact each of these conditions, providing readers with practical insights for their journey towards healing through nutrition.

General Symptoms of Thyroid Imbalances: Thyroid imbalances, whether it's hypothyroidism, hyperthyroidism, or autoimmune conditions like Hashimoto's thyroiditis, can manifest in a variety of symptoms. Here's an overview of the symptoms associated with thyroid imbalances:

- **Fatigue:**
- Feeling excessively tired or lacking energy, even after a good night's sleep.
- **Weight Changes:**
- Unexplained weight gain in hypothyroidism.
- Unintentional weight loss in hyperthyroidism.
- **Temperature Sensitivity:**
- Intolerance to cold in hypothyroidism.
- Heat intolerance and excessive sweating in hyperthyroidism.
- **Mood Changes:**
- Depression, lethargy, or feelings of sadness in hypothyroidism.
- Anxiety, irritability, or nervousness in hyperthyroidism.
- **Heart Rate and Blood Pressure:**
- Bradycardia (slower heart rate) in hypothyroidism.
- Tachycardia (rapid heart rate) and high blood pressure in hyperthyroidism.
- **Skin and Hair Changes:**
- Dry skin, brittle nails, and thinning hair in hypothyroidism.
- Warm, moist skin, and hair loss in hyperthyroidism.
- **Muscle and Joint Discomfort:**
- Muscle aches, stiffness, and joint pain in hypothyroidism.
- Tremors, muscle weakness, and difficulty concentrating in hyperthyroidism.
- **Menstrual Irregularities:**
- Irregular or heavy menstrual periods in hypothyroidism.
- Lighter or irregular periods in hyperthyroidism.

- **Digestive Issues:**
- Constipation in hypothyroidism.
- Diarrhea or more frequent bowel movements in hyperthyroidism.
- **Swelling and Neck Discomfort:**
- Goiter (enlarged thyroid gland) in both hypo- and hyperthyroidism.
- Throat discomfort or a feeling of a lump in the throat (known as a goiter) in both conditions.
- **Sleep Disturbances:**
- Hypothyroidism can lead to excessive sleepiness.
- Hyperthyroidism may cause difficulty falling asleep or staying asleep.

Unique Symptoms for Hashimoto's Thyroiditis:
In addition to the general symptoms, Hashimoto's thyroiditis may present with specific autoimmune-related manifestations, including:

- **Antibody Presence:**
- Presence of antibodies such as thyroid peroxidase antibodies (TPOAb) and thyroglobulin antibodies (TgAb) in blood tests.
- **Fluctuating Symptoms:**
- Symptoms may vary as the autoimmune attack on the thyroid gland fluctuates over time.
- **Thyroid Nodules:**
- Development of nodules or lumps in the thyroid gland.
- **Thyroid Pain:**
- Some individuals may experience pain or discomfort in the thyroid region during flare-ups.

It's important to note that individual experiences can vary, and not everyone with a thyroid imbalance will experience all of these symptoms. If someone suspects they have a thyroid issue, it's crucial to consult with a healthcare professional for proper diagnosis and management.

3

Chapter 2: The Impact of Nutrition on Thyroid Health

U nderstanding the Thyroid-Nutrition Connection

1. Essential Nutrients for Thyroid Function:

i. **Iodine:**

- The role of iodine in thyroid hormone synthesis.
- Dietary sources of iodine and recommended intake.

ii. **Selenium:**

- Selenium's importance in protecting the thyroid gland.
- Selenium-rich foods and supplementation considerations.

iii. **Zinc:**

- Zinc's contribution to thyroid hormone conversion.
- Zinc-rich foods and balancing intake.

iv. **Iron:**

- The impact of iron on thyroid hormone production.
- Iron sources and considerations for absorption.

2. Anti-Inflammatory Foods:

- Exploring the link between inflammation and thyroid health.
- Incorporating anti-inflammatory foods into the diet.
- Recipes and meal ideas featuring anti-inflammatory ingredients.

3. Balancing Macronutrients:
i. Carbohydrates:

- The role of carbohydrates in thyroid hormone production.
- Choosing complex carbohydrates for sustained energy.

ii. Proteins:

- The importance of protein in supporting thyroid function.
- Optimal protein sources for thyroid health.

iii. Fats:

- The impact of healthy fats on hormone regulation.
- Incorporating omega-3 fatty acids for thyroid support.

Foods to Limit or Avoid for Thyroid Health

1. Cruciferous Vegetables:

- Examples: Broccoli, Brussels sprouts, cabbage, cauliflower.
- Why: These vegetables contain compounds known as goitrogens, which can interfere with thyroid function. Cooking may reduce the goitrogenic effect.

2. Soy and Soy Products:

- Examples: Tofu, soy milk, edamame.
- Why: Soy contains goitrogens and can interfere with thyroid hormone absorption. Moderation is key, and cooking or fermenting soy can reduce goitrogen levels.

3. Gluten-Containing Foods:

- Examples: Wheat, barley, rye.
- Why: Some individuals with thyroid disorders, especially those with Hashimoto's, may benefit from reducing or eliminating gluten. Gluten can contribute to inflammation.

4. Processed Foods:

- Examples: Fast food, packaged snacks, sugary treats.
- Why: Processed foods often contain unhealthy fats, excessive salt, and additives that can contribute to inflammation and negatively impact overall health.

5. Excessive Iodine:

- Sources: Iodine supplements, excessive consumption of iodine-rich foods.
- Why: While iodine is essential for thyroid function, excessive intake can lead to thyroid dysfunction, especially in susceptible individuals.

6. Highly Processed Vegetable Oils:

- Examples: Soybean oil, corn oil, canola oil.
- Why: These oils may contribute to inflammation. Opt for healthier fats like olive oil or coconut oil.

7. Foods High in Added Sugar:

- Examples: Sugary beverages, candies, desserts.
- Why: Excessive sugar intake can contribute to inflammation and may negatively impact overall health.

8. Caffeine and Excessive Caffeinated Beverages:

- Sources: Coffee, energy drinks, some teas.
- Why: While moderate caffeine intake is generally fine, excessive amounts can interfere with thyroid hormone absorption and contribute to adrenal stress.

9. Alcohol:

- Why: Alcohol can interfere with the production and utilization of thyroid hormones. Moderation is key.

10. Foods High in Oxalates:

- Examples: Spinach, beet greens, nuts.
- Why: High oxalate levels can interfere with nutrient absorption. Cooking or pairing with calcium-rich foods can mitigate this effect.

11. Excessive Fiber:

- While fiber is generally beneficial, excessive amounts may interfere with the absorption of thyroid medication. It's important to space out fiber intake from medication.

12. Foods with Artificial Trans Fats:

- Examples: Margarine, some packaged snacks.
- Why: Trans fats can contribute to inflammation and have been linked to various health issues.

13. Environmental Contaminants:

- Sources: Certain fish (high in mercury), polluted water.
- Why: Some environmental contaminants can affect thyroid function. Choose fish low in mercury and opt for clean water sources.

14. Non-Organic Produce with High Pesticide Residue:

- Why: Pesticides may disrupt endocrine function, including thyroid health. Choosing organic produce when possible can reduce exposure.

15. Sugary Drinks:

- Examples: Soda, sweetened beverages.
- Why: High sugar content can contribute to inflammation and negatively impact overall health.

16. High-Glycemic Foods:

- Examples: White potatoes, sugary cereals.
- Why: Foods with a high glycemic index can lead to spikes in blood sugar levels, potentially impacting hormonal balance.

17. Low-Calorie or Crash Diets:

- Why: Severely restricting calories or following crash diets can stress the body and negatively affect thyroid function. Encourage a balanced and sustainable approach to nutrition.

18. Unregulated Herbal Supplements:

- Why: Some herbal supplements may interact with thyroid medications or have unknown effects on thyroid function. Always consult with a healthcare professional before taking supplements.

4

Chapter 3: Healing the Thyroid Through Diet

Sample Thyroid-Friendly Diet Plan: Designing a thyroid-friendly diet plan involves incorporating nutrient-rich foods that support thyroid function and avoiding potential triggers. Here's a sample thyroid-friendly diet plan that you can use as a starting point in your daily life;

Day 1: Balanced Start
Breakfast:

- Quinoa Breakfast Bowl:
- Quinoa cooked in almond milk
- Topped with berries, nuts, and a drizzle of honey

Lunch:

- Grilled Chicken Salad:
- Grilled chicken breast
- Mixed greens, cherry tomatoes, cucumbers
- Olive oil and lemon dressing

Snack:

- Greek Yogurt with Walnuts:
- Plain Greek yogurt
- Crushed walnuts for added omega-3s

Dinner:

- Baked Salmon with Roasted Vegetables:

- Baked salmon filet
- Roasted sweet potatoes, broccoli, and carrots
- Quinoa or brown rice on the side

Day 2: Nutrient Boost

Breakfast:

- Green Smoothie:
- Spinach, kale, banana, and a scoop of protein powder
- Blended with almond milk

Lunch:

- Lentil and Vegetable Soup:
- Lentils, carrots, celery, and kale
- Vegetable broth base with herbs and spices

Snack:

- Sliced Apples with Almond Butter:
- Apple slices with a spread of natural almond butter

Dinner:

- Stir-Fried Tofu with Vegetables:
- Tofu stir-fried with bell peppers, broccoli, and snap peas
- Served over quinoa or brown rice

Day 3: Anti-Inflammatory Focus

Breakfast:

- Chia Seed Pudding:
- Chia seeds soaked in coconut milk
- Topped with fresh berries and a sprinkle of hemp seeds

Lunch:

- Salmon and Avocado Wrap:
- Grilled salmon, avocado, and leafy greens
- Whole-grain or gluten-free wrap

Snack:

- Turmeric Golden Milk Smoothie:
- Banana, turmeric, ginger, and a dash of black pepper
- Blended with coconut milk

Dinner:

- Quinoa-Stuffed Bell Peppers:
- Quinoa, black beans, corn, and diced tomatoes
- Baked in bell peppers, topped with salsa

Day 4: Gut Health Emphasis

Breakfast:

- Probiotic-Rich Parfait:

- Greek yogurt with probiotics
- Layered with granola and mixed berries

Lunch:

- Chickpea and Spinach Salad:
- Chickpeas, cherry tomatoes, cucumber, and feta cheese
- Olive oil and lemon dressing

Snack:

- Kimchi with Rice Cakes:
- Fermented kimchi with brown rice cakes

Dinner:

- Chicken Bone Broth Soup:
- Chicken broth with carrots, celery, and kale
- Shredded chicken added for protein

Day 5: Stress Management Integration

Breakfast:

- Oatmeal with Banana and Almonds:
- Rolled oats cooked with almond milk
- Sliced banana and a handful of almonds

Lunch:

- Turkey and Avocado Salad:

- Sliced turkey breast, mixed greens, cherry tomatoes
- Avocado slices with olive oil and balsamic vinegar

Snack:

- Mixed Berries and Dark Chocolate:
- A small portion of mixed berries with a square of dark chocolate

Dinner:

- Baked Cod with Lemon and Herbs:
- Cod fillet seasoned with lemon and herbs
- Steamed asparagus and quinoa on the side

Key Considerations:

- Encourage hydration with water, herbal teas, and coconut water.
- Emphasize portion control for balanced energy throughout the day.
- Tailor the plan to individual dietary preferences, allergies, and sensitivities.
- Advise readers to consult with a healthcare professional or dietitian before making significant changes to their diet.

Feel free to customize this sample diet plan to suit the preferences and dietary needs of yours. Providing a variety of nutrient-dense, thyroid-supportive options will help you embark on a journey towards healing through nutrition.

Healing the Thyroid Through Diet - Vegetarian Edition

Some Sample Thyroid-Friendly Vegetarian Diet Plan

Day 1: Wholesome Start

Breakfast:

- Masala Oats:
- Oats cooked with turmeric, cumin, mustard seeds, and mixed vegetables
- Topped with chopped coriander and a squeeze of lemon

Lunch:

- Chickpea Spinach Curry:
- Chickpeas and spinach cooked in a tomato-based curry
- Served with brown rice or whole wheat roti

Snack:

- Cucumber and Hummus:
- Sliced cucumber with homemade hummus

Dinner:

- Paneer Tikka Salad:
- Grilled paneer (Indian cottage cheese) marinated in spices
- Tossed with mixed greens, tomatoes, and bell peppers

Day 2: Plant-Powered Nutrients

Breakfast:

- Smoothie Bowl:
- Blended banana, mango, spinach, and a scoop of plant-based protein powder
- Topped with chia seeds, flaxseeds, and fresh berries

Lunch:

- Dal Tadka with Quinoa:
- Yellow lentils cooked with spices, topped with a tempering of cumin and mustard seeds
- Served with quinoa

Snack:

- Roasted Chickpeas:
- Chickpeas roasted with chaat masala and cumin

Dinner:

- Stuffed Bell Peppers with Brown Rice:
- Bell peppers stuffed with spiced brown rice, black beans, and corn
- Baked until tender

Day 3: Ayurvedic Flavors

Breakfast:

- Upma:
- Semolina cooked with mustard seeds, curry leaves, and vegetables
- Garnished with chopped cilantro and grated coconut

Lunch:

- Rajma (Kidney Beans) and Quinoa:
- Rajma cooked in a tomato-based curry
- Served with quinoa

Snack:

- Yogurt with Turmeric and Almonds:
- Plain yogurt mixed with turmeric and topped with sliced almonds

Dinner:

- Vegetable Biryani:
- Fragrant basmati rice cooked with mixed vegetables and biryani spices

Day 4: Probiotic Delights

Breakfast:

- Poha:
- Flattened rice cooked with mustard seeds, turmeric, and peanuts

- Garnished with fresh coriander and a squeeze of lime

Lunch:

- Palak (Spinach) and Tofu Curry:
- Tofu and spinach cooked in a coconut milk-based curry
- Served with quinoa or whole wheat roti

Snack:

- Kokum and Mint Cooler:
- Kokum-infused drink with fresh mint leaves

Dinner:

- Vegetarian Kofta Curry:
- Vegetable koftas in a rich tomato-based curry
- Served with brown rice

Day 5: Balanced Energizers

Breakfast:

- Idli with Sambar and Coconut Chutney:
- Steamed rice cakes served with lentil-based sambar and coconut chutney

Lunch:

- Masoor Dal with Quinoa:
- Masoor dal (red lentils) cooked with spices

- Served with quinoa

Snack:

- Dhokla:
- Steamed fermented cakes made from gram flour
- Served with mint chutney

Dinner:

- Vegetable Stir-Fry with Millets:
- Mixed vegetables stir-fried with tofu and tossed with cooked millets

Key Considerations:

- Utilize local and seasonal produce for freshness and variety.
- Include a mix of pulses, legumes, and plant-based protein sources.
- Adjust spice levels according to individual preferences.
- Encourage regular hydration with water, herbal teas, and fresh coconut water.

This vegetarian thyroid-friendly diet plan integrates traditional Indian flavors and ingredients while providing essential nutrients to support thyroid health. As always, advise readers to consult with a healthcare professional or dietitian before making significant changes to their diet.

5

Chapter 4: Lifestyle Changes for Thyroid Health

Addressing lifestyle changes is crucial for holistic thyroid health. Here's a comprehensive guide for your thyroid health :

1. Stress Management Techniques:

a. Mindfulness Meditation:

- How it Helps: Reduces cortisol levels, promotes relaxation, and enhances overall well-being.
- Implementation: Guide through simple mindfulness meditation exercises.

b. Deep Breathing Exercises:

- How it Helps: Activates the relaxation response, lowers stress hormones, and improves oxygenation.
- Implementation: Learn deep breathing techniques, such as diaphragmatic breathing or box breathing, for quick stress relief.

c. Yoga for Thyroid Health:

- How it Helps: Combines physical postures, breath control, and meditation to reduce stress and enhance hormonal balance.
- Implementation: beginner-friendly yoga routine focusing on poses beneficial for thyroid health.

d. Journaling for Emotional Release:

- How it Helps: Allows individuals to express and process emotions, reducing emotional stress.
- Implementation: Maintain a gratitude journal or expressive journaling for emotional well-being.

e. Adaptogenic Herbs:

- How it Helps: Certain herbs like ashwagandha and holy basil can help the body adapt to stress.
- Implementation: Incorporating adaptogenic herbs into the diet, whether through teas, supplements, or culinary uses.

2. Importance of Quality Sleep for Thyroid Function:

a. Sleep and Hormonal Regulation:

- Why Quality Sleep Matters: Sleep influences the secretion of hormones, including thyroid hormones.
- Tips for Quality Sleep: Establish a consistent sleep schedule, create a relaxing bedtime routine, and optimize sleep environment.

b. Blue Light Reduction:

- How it Helps: Exposure to blue light from screens can disrupt melatonin production, affecting sleep.
- Implementation: Limiting screen time before bedtime or using blue light filters on electronic devices are way to go.

c. Sleep Hygiene Practices:

- Creating a Sleep-Inducing Environment: Dark, cool, and quiet rooms promote restful sleep.
- Bedtime Rituals: Calming activities before bedtime, such as reading or gentle stretching must be adopted for bedtime rituals.

d. Herbal Teas for Sleep:

- Relaxing Botanicals: Chamomile, valerian root, and lavender can promote relaxation and aid in sleep.
- Incorporation: Herbal teas are recommended here as part of a calming bedtime routine.

3. Exercise and its Impact on Thyroid Health:

a. Cardiovascular Exercise:

- How it Helps: Boosts metabolism, improves blood flow, and supports overall thyroid function.
- Recommendations: Moderate-intensity activities like brisk walking, cycling, or swimming.

b. Strength Training:

- How it Helps: Builds muscle mass, which can enhance metabolism and support weight management.
- Guidelines: Include resistance training exercises using body weight, dumbbells, or resistance bands.

c. Yoga and Tai Chi:

- How it Helps: Combines movement, breath, and mindfulness, promoting relaxation and balance.
- Incorporation: Incorporating yoga or tai chi sessions into the weekly routine are suggested.

d. Interval Training:

- How it Helps: High-intensity intervals can improve cardiovascular health and metabolic rate.
- Cautions: Moderation is key, especially for individuals with thyroid disorders, and recommend consulting a fitness professional.

e. *Outdoor Activities:*

- The Role of Sunlight: Exposure to natural light can regulate circadian rhythms and positively impact mood.
- Suggestions: Outdoor activities like walking or jogging in a park are advised.

Key Considerations:

This chapter provides a holistic approach, addressing stress management, quality sleep, and exercise, essential components for supporting thyroid health. Readers can use these practical tips to enhance their daily routines and promote overall wellness.

6

Chapter 5: Herbal Support and Supplements for Thyroid Health

Overview of Herbs Supporting Thyroid Health:

1. Ashwagandha (Withania somnifera):

- Adaptogenic Properties: Ashwagandha is an adaptogenic herb that helps the body adapt to stress.
- Thyroid Function: Studies suggest it may help balance thyroid hormones, particularly in cases of stress-induced thyroid imbalances.

2. Holy Basil (Ocimum sanctum or Tulsi):

- Adaptogenic and Antioxidant: Holy Basil is an adaptogen with antioxidant properties.
- Anti-Inflammatory Effects: Supports thyroid health by reducing inflammation and oxidative stress.

3. Bladderwrack (Fucus vesiculosus):

- Rich in Iodine: Contains iodine, essential for thyroid hormone production.
- Supports Thyroid Function: May assist in maintaining healthy thyroid function, but caution is advised due to potential iodine excess.

4. Eleuthero (Eleutherococcus senticosus):

- Adaptogenic Properties: Similar to ashwagandha, eleuthero helps the body adapt to stress.
- Energy and Vitality: Supports overall energy levels and may assist in managing fatigue associated with thyroid disorders.

5. Coleus Forskohlii:

- Forskolin Content: Forskolin, derived from the root, has shown potential benefits for thyroid health.
- Cyclic AMP Activation: May enhance the production of cyclic AMP, which plays a role in thyroid hormone synthesis.

6. Guggul (Commiphora wightii):

- Anti-Inflammatory: Known for its anti-inflammatory properties.
- Thyroid Hormone Conversion: May support the conversion of T4 to the active T3 form.

7. Dandelion Root (Taraxacum officinale):

- Liver Support: Supports liver health, which is crucial for thyroid hormone conversion.
- Rich in Nutrients: Provides vitamins and minerals that contribute to overall well-being.

8. Turmeric (Curcuma longa):

- Anti-Inflammatory and Antioxidant: Turmeric's active compound, curcumin, has anti-inflammatory and antioxidant effects.
- Thyroid and Autoimmunity: May be beneficial in managing thyroid disorders with autoimmune components.

9. Nettle (Urtica dioica):

- Rich in Nutrients: Nettle is rich in vitamins and minerals, including iodine.
- Thyroid Support: May help support overall thyroid health.

10. Spirulina:

- Nutrient-Rich: Spirulina is a nutrient-dense algae.
- Iodine Content: Contains iodine and other nutrients important for thyroid function.

Important Considerations:

- Consultation with Healthcare Professionals: Emphasize the importance of consulting healthcare professionals before incorporating herbs or supplements, especially if individuals are on medication.

- Quality of Supplements: Encourage readers to choose high-quality supplements from reputable sources to ensure purity and effectiveness.
- Individual Responses: Acknowledge that individuals may respond differently to herbs, and it's essential to monitor how their bodies react.
- Balanced Approach: Herbs can complement lifestyle changes but should not replace a balanced diet, stress management, and other healthy habits.

Note: Readers are always advised to consult with a healthcare professional or a qualified herbalist before introducing new herbs or supplements, especially if they are already on medication or have pre-existing health conditions.

Here are some herbs that are commonly found in India and are known for their potential benefits in supporting thyroid health:

1. Ashwagandha (Withania somnifera):

- Overview: An adaptogenic herb, commonly used in Ayurveda.
- Benefits: Supports the body's response to stress, may help balance thyroid hormones.

2. Holy Basil (Tulsi - Ocimum sanctum):

- Overview: Revered in Ayurveda for its medicinal properties.
- Benefits: Acts as an adaptogen, reduces inflammation, and supports overall well-being.

3. Bladderwrack (Sargassum):

- Overview: A type of seaweed commonly found in coastal areas.
- Benefits: Rich in iodine, which is crucial for thyroid function.

4. Guggul (Commiphora wightii):

- Overview: Resin obtained from the mukul myrrh tree.
- Benefits: Known for its anti-inflammatory properties and potential support for thyroid function.

5. Turmeric (Curcuma longa):

- Overview: Widely used in Indian cuisine and traditional medicine.
- Benefits: Contains curcumin, which has anti-inflammatory and antioxidant effects.

6. Nettle (Urtica dioica):

- Overview: Commonly found in India and used in traditional medicine.
- Benefits: Rich in vitamins and minerals, including iodine, supporting thyroid health.

7. Triphala:

- Overview: A combination of three fruits - Amalaki, Bibhitaki, and Haritaki.
- Benefits: Supports digestion, detoxification, and overall health, indirectly impacting thyroid function.

8. Brahmi (Bacopa monnieri):

- Overview: Adaptogenic herb used in Ayurveda.
- Benefits: Supports cognitive function, may help manage stress.

9. Spirulina:

- Overview: Blue-green algae cultivated in certain regions of India.
- Benefits: Nutrient-dense, contains iodine and other essential nutrients.

10. Amla (Indian Gooseberry):

- Overview: Rich in vitamin C and antioxidants.
- Benefits: Supports immune function and overall well-being.

11. Cumin (Cuminum cyminum):

- Overview: Commonly used spice in Indian cooking.
- Benefits: Supports digestion and may have anti-inflammatory properties.

12. Coriander (Coriandrum sativum):

- Overview: Widely used herb in Indian cuisine.
- Benefits: Contains antioxidants and may have anti-inflammatory effects.

13. Fenugreek (Trigonella foenum-graecum):

- Overview: Seeds commonly used in Indian cooking.
- Benefits: Supports digestion and may have anti-inflammatory properties.

14. Trikatu:

- Overview: A blend of three spices - ginger, black pepper, and long pepper.
- Benefits: Supports digestion and metabolism.

15. Ajwain (Carom Seeds - Trachyspermum ammi):

- Overview: Seeds commonly used in Indian cuisine.
- Benefits: Supports digestion and may have antimicrobial properties.

Important Considerations:

- Dosage and Duration: Always follow recommended dosages and consult with healthcare professionals, especially if considering long-term use.
- Individual Responses: Herbs may affect individuals differently, so it's important to monitor their impact on personal health.
- Incorporation in Diet: Many of these herbs and spices can be easily incorporated into daily cooking for added flavor and potential health benefits.

Important Considerations:

- Consultation with Healthcare Professionals: Before starting any supplements, individuals should consult with their healthcare provider to ensure the supplements are appropriate for their specific health needs.
- Individual Needs: Supplement needs vary based on individual health conditions, deficiencies, and overall diet.
- Monitoring Levels: Regular monitoring of nutrient levels through blood tests can help ensure that supplementation is adequate but not excessive.
- Quality of Supplements: Choose high-quality supplements from reputable brands to ensure purity and potency.

"It's crucial for individuals to work closely with healthcare professionals, including endocrinologists and registered dietitians, to determine the right supplements based on their unique health circumstances. Supplements should complement a well-balanced diet and lifestyle modifications rather than serve as a primary or sole intervention."

Chapter 6: Gut Health and Thyroid Connection

Understanding the Link Between Gut Health and Thyroid Function: "Exploring the connection between gut health and thyroid function is an important aspect of holistic wellness."

The Gut-Thyroid Axis:

- **Overview:** Imagine your gut and thyroid as inseparable friends in a constant exchange of messages. This dynamic duo forms the Gut-Thyroid Axis, a two-way communication system that orchestrates the harmony of your body.
- **Key Points:**
- **Microbiome Influence:** Envision your gut as a thriving city, bustling with microbial activity. These inhabitants play a crucial role in converting inactive thyroid hormones into their active forms, ensuring optimal thyroid function.
- Nutrient Absorption: Picture the gut as the thyroid's diligent assistant, ensuring the absorption of essential nutrients like iodine, crucial for thyroid health.

L eaky Gut and Autoimmunity:

- **Overview:** Picture your gut as a fortress defending your body against invaders. But what if there are tiny breaches in its walls? This is what we call a leaky gut, potentially triggering an autoimmune response against the thyroid.
  - **Key Points:**
  - **Intestinal Permeability:** Visualize the gut lining as a drawbridge; when it's lowered, unwanted invaders like undigested food particles can sneak in, causing havoc.

- **Autoimmune Thyroid Conditions:** Envision your immune system as a vigilant guard, mistakenly attacking the thyroid due to the confusion caused by the leaky gut.

Probiotics and Digestive Health:

Role of Probiotics:

- **Overview**: Introduce yourselves to the superheroes of gut health – probiotics. These friendly bacteria are like the peacekeepers of a microbial city, ensuring harmony within.
- **Key Points:**
- **Microbiome Diversity:** Picture probiotics as event organizers throwing a lively party in your gut, fostering a diverse and harmonious microbial community.
- **Anti-Inflammatory Effects:** Envision probiotics as skilled firefighters, calming down inflammation and creating a peaceful environment within your gut.

Probiotics and Thyroid Health:

- **Overview:** Probiotics go beyond gut peacekeeping; they extend their support to the thyroid. Visualize them as helpful neighbors contributing to the overall well-being of your body.
- **Key Points:**
- **Regulation of Inflammation**: Imagine probiotics as skilled negotiators, helping to cool down inflammation and creating a thyroid-friendly atmosphere.
- **Immunomodulatory Effects**: Picture probiotics as diplomats maintaining a healthy relationship between the immune system and the thyroid.

Sources of Probiotics:

- **Overview**: Now, let's explore how to recruit these friendly allies into your system. Your kitchen becomes a recruitment center for probiotics.
- **Key Points:**
- **Fermented Foods**: Enlist fermented foods like yogurt, sauerkraut, and kimchi as your probiotic army, ready to support your gut health.
- **Probiotic Supplements**: Consider these as reinforcements, ensuring a robust microbial defense when your gut needs an extra boost.

Strategies for Improving Gut Health:

1. **Balanced Diet**:

- **Overview**: Visualize your plate as a banquet, offering a variety of nutrient-rich dishes to nourish your gut inhabitants. It's time to throw a feast for the microbial community within you.
- **Key Points**:
- **Fiber Intake**: Imagine fiber as the VIP dish, attracting a diverse crowd of friendly microbes to the banquet. A rich and varied diet keeps your gut community happy and thriving.
- **Hydration**: Visualize water as the drink of choice at your banquet, ensuring your microbial citizens are happily hydrated and flourishing.

2. **Prebiotics:**

- **Overview**: It's not just about the guests; we need to keep them well-fed too. Prebiotics are like the banquet organizers, ensuring

everyone has something to munch on.
- **Key Points**:
- **Natural Sources**: Picture garlic, onions, and bananas as the prebiotic chefs creating a delectable menu for your gut residents. Dietary fiber acts as the red carpet guiding prebiotics to their VIP destination.

3. **Avoiding Gut Irritants**:

- **Overview**: Protect your gut from troublemakers. Visualize your gut as a peaceful neighborhood, and avoiding irritants is like maintaining the tranquility within.
- **Key Points**:
- **Processed Foods**: Imagine processed foods as troublemakers, stirring up chaos in the gut community. Opt for whole, unprocessed foods to maintain peace and order.
- **Potential Allergens**: Identify potential allergens as trespassers and take measures to keep them out, ensuring the security of your gut community.

4. **Managing Stress**:

- **Overview**: Now, let's create a serene environment for your gut inhabitants. Imagine stress management as a relaxation retreat, providing your gut citizens with a stress-free zone to thrive.
- **Key Points**:
- **Mind-Body Techniques**: Picture mindfulness and deep breathing as calming activities, offering your gut inhabitants moments of peace and tranquility.
- **Regular Physical Activity**: Visualize physical activity as a community event, bringing joy and balance to the gut neighborhood,

keeping the microbial community vibrant and alive.

5. Proactive Lifestyle Choices:

- **Overview:** It's time for your gut citizens to thrive. Visualize a thriving community with everyone actively participating in the well-being of the neighborhood.
- **Key Points**:
- **Adequate Sleep**: Picture sleep as the nightly rejuvenation for your gut inhabitants, ensuring their vitality and health.
- **Regular Movement**: Visualize regular movement as a celebration, keeping the gut community vibrant, active, and flourishing.

Key Considerations for Readers:

- **Gradual Changes:** readers are encouraged to make small, gradual changes, allowing their gut community to adapt and thrive over time.
- **Individual Variability:** everyone's gut is unique, and responses to changes may vary. It's okay to experiment and find what works best for you.
- **Seeking Professional Guidance:**. A healthcare professional can provide tailored recommendations based on individual health conditions and needs, therefore the importance of consulting healthcare professionals for personalized advice on gut health strategies is emphasized here.

"In this detailed exploration, we've painted a vivid picture of the intricate Gut Health and Thyroid Connection. Readers are invited to visualize their own

bodies as dynamic ecosystems, where the choices they make play a crucial role in fostering a thriving and harmonious environment. Through relatable metaphors and practical tips, readers are empowered to take charge of their gut health, ultimately supporting their thyroid function and overall well-being."

8

Chapter 7: Mind-Body Connection

Unlocking the Harmony Within:

Overview:

- **Imagine Your Body as an Orchestra**: Envision your body as a symphony where each organ and system plays a unique instrument. The mind conducts this orchestra, creating a harmonious melody of well-being.
  - **Key Message:** The mind and body are interconnected, each influencing the other's rhythm, creating a profound symphony of health.

Metaphors to Illuminate the Mind-Body Connection:

1. **The Captain and the Ship:**

- **Visualize Your Mind as the Captain**: Picture your mind as the captain steering a ship, navigating the vast seas of your body. The body, the ship, responds to the captain's commands, showcasing the powerful influence of your thoughts on physical well-being.

- **Key Message**: Your thoughts guide the course of your body, illustrating the intimate connection between mental states and physical responses.

2. **The Garden and the Gardener**:

- **Envision Your Mind as the Gardener:** Imagine your mind as the diligent gardener tending to the garden of your body. Thoughts, like seeds, sprout into emotions and actions, shaping the overall landscape of your well-being.
- **Key Message**: Cultivating positive thoughts nurtures a flourishing garden of health, emphasizing the impact of mental well-being on physical vitality.

3. **The Weaver and the Tapestry**:

- **See Your Mind as the Weaver**: Visualize your mind as a skilled weaver crafting a vibrant tapestry. Each thought, emotion, and action weaves together to form the intricate design of your body's health.
- **Key Message**: The mind weaves the fabric of your physical well-being, highlighting the interconnectedness of mental and physical aspects.

Exploration of Mind-Body Practices:

1. **Meditation as the Mind's Serenade**:

- **Overview**: Picture meditation as a soothing serenade for the mind, a melody that resonates throughout your body. Through mindfulness, the mind calms the orchestra, promoting harmony within.

- **Key Benefits**: Stress reduction, improved focus, and a sense of inner peace.

2. Exercise as the Body's Dance:

- **Overview**: Envision exercise as a lively dance for the body, a rhythmic movement that echoes the energy of the mind. The dance fosters a joyous connection between mental and physical vitality.
- **Key Benefits**: Enhanced mood, increased energy, and improved overall well-being.

3. Breathwork as the Harmony Between Mind and Body:

- **Overview:** See breathwork as the harmonious breath shared between the mind and body. Inhales and exhales become the synchronized dance, fostering a deep connection and balance.
- **Key Benefits**: Stress relief, improved respiratory function, and a heightened sense of awareness.

4. Visualization as the Architect of Wellness:

- **Overview**: Imagine visualization as the architectural blueprint crafted by the mind. Detailed mental images shape the physical landscape, creating a vision of health and vitality.
- **Key Benefits**: Enhanced motivation, goal attainment, and a positive impact on physical well-being.

Cultivate the Mind-Body Connection:

1. The Daily Symphony:

- **Overview**: readers are encouraged to view their daily routines as a symphony, with each mindful choice contributing to the harmonious melody of well-being. Small, intentional actions shape the overall composition.
- **Key Message**: Every thought, action, and choice plays a part in the daily symphony of mind-body connection.

2. Emotional Gardening:

- **Overview**: Get inspired to engage in emotional gardening, tending to their thoughts and feelings. Nurturing positivity and mindfulness creates a fertile ground for holistic well-being.
- **Key Message**: Like a garden, the mind flourishes with intentional care and cultivation.

3. Weaving a Tapestry of Health:

- **Overview**: Guide yourself to actively participate in weaving the tapestry of your health. Each positive thought and action contributes to the vibrant fabric of overall well-being.
- **Key Message**: Wellness is a conscious creation, and you are the weavers of your health tapestry.

<u>Key Considerations for Readers</u>:

"In this exploration of the Mind-Body Connection, readers are invited to envision their bodies as intricate symphonies, gardens, and tapestries. Metaphors provide a tangible way to grasp the profound interplay between the mind and body, while practical practices empower readers to actively cultivate a harmonious relationship for holistic well-being."

Yoga Asanas for Mind-Body Connection:

Including accessible yoga asanas in your daily life on the mind-body connection is a wonderful thing. Here are descriptions of some beginner-friendly yoga poses that can be practiced easily at home:

1. **Mountain Pose (Tadasana):**

- Stand tall with feet together, arms by your sides. Reach your arms overhead, palms facing each other.
- **Benefits**: Improves posture, increases awareness of body alignment, and promotes a sense of grounding.

2. **Tree Pose (Vrikshasana):**

- Stand on one leg, place the sole of the other foot on the inner thigh or calf, and bring your palms together in front of your chest.
- Benefits: Enhances balance, concentration, and mental focus, fostering a connection between mind and body.

3. **Child's Pose (Balasana):**

- Kneel on the mat, sit back on your heels, and reach your arms forward, lowering your chest towards the floor.

- **Benefits**: Relieves stress, calms the mind, and stretches the back, promoting a sense of relaxation.

4. Downward Facing Dog (Adho Mukha Svanasana):

- Start on your hands and knees, lift your hips towards the ceiling, straighten your legs, and press your heels towards the floor.
- **Benefits**: Strengthens the entire body, stretches the spine, and energizes the mind.

5. Warrior I (Virabhadrasana I):

- Step one foot back, bend the front knee, and extend your arms overhead, palms facing each other.
- **Benefits**: Builds strength in the legs, opens the chest, and instills a sense of inner strength.

6. Seated Forward Bend (Paschimottanasana):

- Sit with legs extended, hinge at the hips, and reach towards your toes, keeping your back straight.
- **Benefits**: Stretches the spine and hamstrings, calms the mind, and promotes introspection.

7. Corpse Pose (Savasana):

- Lie on your back, arms by your sides, and legs extended. Close your eyes and focus on your breath.
- **Benefits**: Relaxes the entire body, reduces stress, and enhances the mind-body connection through mindfulness.

Tips for Practicing Yoga at Home:

- *Start Slow: If you're new to yoga, begin with a few poses and gradually add more as you become comfortable.*
- *Listen to Your Body: Pay attention to how your body feels during each pose. If something doesn't feel right, modify or skip it.*
- *Use Props: Bolsters, blocks, and straps can aid in proper alignment and make the poses more accessible.*
- *Combine with Mindfulness: As you move through the poses, focus on your breath*

9

Chapter 8: Thyroid-Friendly Recipes

In this chapter, we embark on a culinary journey that aligns with the recommended diet for thyroid health. These recipes are thoughtfully curated to include ingredients known for their positive impact on thyroid function. Embracing a nutrient-rich and balanced approach, these dishes aim to support your well-being and nourish your body.

1. Quinoa and Vegetable Buddha Bowl:

Ingredients:

```
Quinoa
Mixed vegetables (broccoli, carrots, bell peppers)
Chickpeas
Avocado
Spinach
```

Instructions:

Cook quinoa according to package instructions.
Roast mixed vegetables and chickpeas in olive oil and your
favorite spices.
Assemble the bowl with a base of quinoa, topped with roasted
vegetables, chickpeas, sliced avocado, and fresh spinach.

2. Salmon and Kale Salad:

Ingredients:

Grilled salmon fillet
Kale leaves
Cherry tomatoes
Cucumber
Olive oil and lemon dressing

Instructions:

Grill salmon with a sprinkle of sea salt and black pepper.
Massage kale leaves with olive oil to soften.
Combine grilled salmon, kale, cherry tomatoes, and cucumber.
Drizzle with olive oil and lemon dressing.

3. Sweet Potato and Lentil Soup:

Ingredients:

Sweet potatoes
Red lentils
Onion
Garlic

Vegetable broth

Instructions:

Sauté onions and garlic in olive oil until golden.
Add diced sweet potatoes, red lentils, and vegetable broth.
Simmer until sweet potatoes and lentils are tender. Blend to
your desired consistency.

4. Quinoa-Stuffed Bell Peppers:

Ingredients:

Bell peppers
Quinoa
Black beans
Corn
Diced tomatoes

Instructions:

Cook quinoa and mix with black beans, corn, and diced
tomatoes.
Cut bell peppers in half, removing seeds. Stuff with quinoa
mixture.
Bake until peppers are tender.

5. Greek Yogurt and Berry Parfait:

Ingredients:

```
Greek yogurt
Mixed berries (blueberries, strawberries, raspberries)
Granola
Honey
```

Instructions:

```
Layer Greek yogurt with mixed berries in a glass.
Top with granola for crunch.
Drizzle honey over the parfait for sweetness.
```

Tips for Thyroid-Friendly Cooking:

- Incorporate Iodine-Rich Foods: Include seafood, dairy(prefer plant based milk), and iodized salt to support thyroid function.
- Prioritize Selenium: Foods like Brazil nuts, sunflower seeds, and eggs are excellent sources of selenium, beneficial for thyroid health.
- Embrace Anti-Inflammatory Ingredients: Incorporate ginger, turmeric, and fatty fish to help reduce inflammation.

These recipes are designed not only to cater to the specific needs of thyroid health but also to tantalize your taste buds. Enjoy these delicious and nourishing dishes as part of your journey towards a thyroid-friendly lifestyle

10

Chapter 9: Overcoming Challenges

As you embark on the transformative journey of healing your thyroid through lifestyle and dietary changes, it's essential to address the common obstacles that may arise along the way. In this chapter, we will explore these challenges and equip ourselves with effective strategies to overcome them, ensuring we stay on track towards a healthier and balanced life.

Common Obstacles in Implementing Lifestyle and Dietary Changes:

1. **Resistance to Change**:

- **Description**: The comfort of familiar habits can create resistance to change. Breaking away from routine may initially feel challenging.
- **Strategy: Gradual Transition:** Implement changes slowly, allowing your mind and body to adapt. Start with small adjustments and gradually progress to more significant transformations.

2. **Social and Cultural Influences**:

- **Description**: Social gatherings and cultural practices may involve foods or habits that don't align with your new lifestyle.
- **Strategy**: Communicate your dietary preferences to friends and family. Plan ahead for social events by suggesting alternative food options or bringing your own thyroid-friendly dish.

3. **Overwhelm and Information Overload**:

- **Description**: The abundance of information on thyroid health can be overwhelming, leading to confusion and uncertainty.
- **Strategy**: Guided Learning - Seek guidance from reliable sources or healthcare professionals. Create a personalized plan based on your specific needs, making the journey more manageable.

Strategies for Overcoming Challenges and Staying on Track:

1. **Mindful Awareness**:

- **Description**: Develop awareness of your thoughts, feelings, and behaviors related to lifestyle changes.
- **Strategy**: Journaling - Keep a journal to track your progress, emotions, and challenges. Reflecting on your journey fosters mindfulness and helps you make informed decisions.

2. **Community Support**:

- **Description**: Sharing your journey with like-minded individuals creates a supportive environment.

- **Strategy**: Join Support Groups - Connect with online or local support groups focused on thyroid health. Share experiences, seek advice, and celebrate successes together.

3. **Flexibility in Planning**:

- **Description**: Rigidity in planning can lead to frustration when unexpected situations arise.
- **Strategy**: Flexible Approach - Embrace flexibility in your plans. Life is dynamic, and adjustments may be necessary. Have alternative strategies for different situations.

4. **Celebrate Small Wins**:

- **Description**: Acknowledge and celebrate your achievements, no matter how small.
- **Strategy**: Reward System - Establish a reward system for reaching milestones. Treat yourself with something enjoyable when you accomplish a goal, fostering motivation.

5. **Professional Guidance**:

- **Description**: Navigating health challenges can be complex; seeking professional advice is crucial.
- **Strategy**: Consultation with Experts - Regularly consult healthcare professionals, nutritionists, or wellness experts. Their guidance ensures your approach aligns with your unique health requirements.

6. **Self-Compassion**:

- **Description**: Negative self-talk can hinder progress and erode motivation.

- **Strategy**: Positive Affirmations - Practice positive affirmations to cultivate self-compassion. Remind yourself that this journey is about progress, not perfection.

"Overcoming challenges is an integral part of any transformative process. By recognizing common obstacles and implementing effective strategies, you empower yourself to navigate the complexities of lifestyle and dietary changes with resilience and determination. Remember, each step forward is a victory on your path to thyroid health and overall well-being."

11

Chapter 10: Personal Stories of Healing

In the final chapter of our journey together, we delve into the inspiring narratives of individuals who have triumphed over thyroid health challenges through dedicated nutrition and lifestyle changes. These real-life success stories offer a beacon of hope, proving that transformation is not only possible but achievable through perseverance, resilience, and a commitment to holistic well-being.

Unveiling Triumphs:

1. Ananya's Thyroid Transformation:

- **Background:** Ananya, a 35-year-old professional from Mumbai, faced the challenges of hypothyroidism, leading to persistent fatigue and weight gain.
- **Transformation:** Embracing a balanced diet rich in iodine and selenium, Ananya incorporated traditional Indian superfoods like seaweed, nuts, and lentils. Regular yoga and meditation became integral to her routine, contributing to improved energy levels and weight management.

2. Raj's Journey to Balance:

- **Background:** Raj, a 40-year-old entrepreneur from Delhi, navigated the complexities of hyperthyroidism, disrupting his busy work schedule.
- **Transformation:** Raj adopted a personalized approach, modifying his dietary habits by incorporating more cooling foods like cucumber, mint, and coconut water. He embraced Ayurvedic practices, including regular consumption of ashwagandha, which played a pivotal role in managing stress and supporting his thyroid health.

3. Priya's Holistic Healing with Ayurveda:

- **Background:** Priya, a 30-year-old mother from Chennai, grappled with Hashimoto's thyroiditis, experiencing fluctuations in mood and energy levels.
- **Transformation:** Priya turned to Ayurveda, incorporating ghee, turmeric, and triphala into her diet. Daily practices of pranayama and mindfulness became her anchors, contributing to a holistic approach that addressed both physical and mental well-being.

"These examples are inspired by the rich cultural and dietary diversity present in India. They highlight how individuals from different regions and backgrounds can draw on traditional practices and regional foods to support their thyroid health through nutrition and lifestyle changes. The key takeaway is the adaptability of these approaches to suit the unique needs and cultural contexts of individuals on their healing journeys."

12

Conclusion

Key Takeaways:

*A*s we conclude this insightful journey into understanding and healing thyroid health through nutrition and lifestyle changes, let's recap the key takeaways that can empower you on your path to thyroid wellness:

- **Mind-Body Connection**: Recognize the profound interplay between your thoughts, emotions, and physical well-being. Cultivating a harmonious mind-body connection is foundational to thyroid health.
- **Nutrient-Rich Diet:** Prioritize foods rich in iodine, selenium, and anti-inflammatory properties. Embrace a balanced diet that includes a variety of fruits, vegetables, lean proteins, and whole grains.
- **Lifestyle Choices**: Integrate stress management techniques, regular exercise, and quality sleep into your daily routine. These lifestyle choices contribute significantly to supporting thyroid function.

- **Individualized Approach:** Your journey is unique, and so are your needs. Tailor nutrition and lifestyle changes to align with your specific health requirements, seeking guidance from healthcare professionals when needed.
- **Celebrate Progress:** Acknowledge and celebrate every step forward, no matter how small. Progress is a continuous journey, and each positive change contributes to your overall well-being.

Take Proactive Steps for Their Thyroid Health:

As you close this chapter and embark on the next phase of your health journey, I encourage you to take proactive steps for your thyroid health:

- **Empower Yourself with Knowledge:** Stay informed about thyroid health, nutrition, and lifestyle choices. Knowledge is a powerful tool that enables you to make informed decisions for your well-being.
- **Build a Support System:** Surround yourself with a supportive network of friends, family, and healthcare professionals. Share your goals and challenges, seeking guidance and encouragement along the way.
- **Set Realistic Goals:** Establish achievable goals and milestones on your path to thyroid wellness. Break down larger objectives into smaller, manageable steps, celebrating your accomplishments at each stage.
- **Embrace Consistency:** The journey to thyroid health is a marathon, not a sprint. Embrace consistency in your efforts, understanding that lasting changes take time. Be patient with yourself and stay committed to your well-being.
- **Listen to Your Body:** Pay attention to the signals your body provides. Tune in to how specific foods, activities, and lifestyle

choices impact your overall health. Your body is a unique guide on your journey to wellness.

Remember, this book is not just an end but a beginning – a starting point for you to take control of your thyroid health and lead a life filled with vitality and balance. Your story of healing is waiting to unfold, and by taking proactive steps today, you are paving the way for a healthier and more vibrant tomorrow.

Wishing you a journey filled with discovery, empowerment, and the radiant well-being you deserve.

With warm regards,

Richa Yadav

Author, "Nourish Your Thyroid: A Guide to Healing through Nutrition and Lifestyle"

13

Resources

ttps://www.ncbi.nlm.nih.gov/pmc/articles/PMC5307254/
https://academic.oup.com/qjmed/article/95/9/559/1574610?login=false

Malik, R., & Hodgson, H. J. F. (2002b). The relationship between the thyroid gland and the liver. *Heal Your Thyroid With Nutrition, 95*(9), 559–569. https://doi.org/10.1093/qjmed/95.9.559

https://pubmed.ncbi.nlm.nih.gov/36909313/

Benítes-Zapata, V. A., Ignacio-Cconchoy, F. L., Ulloque-Badaracco, J. R., Hernández-Bustamante, E. A., Alarcón-Braga, E. A., Al-kassab-Córdova, A., & Herrera-Añazco, P. (2023). Vitamin B12 levels in thyroid disorders: A systematic review and meta-analysis. *Frontiers in Endocrinology, 14.* https://doi.org/10.3389/fendo.2023.1070592

https://pubmed.ncbi.nlm.nih.gov/12205333/

Malik, R., & Hodgson, H. J. F. (2002). The relationship between the thyroid gland and the liver. *Healing Thyroid With Nutrition, 95*(9), 559–569. https://doi.org/10.1093/qjmed/95.9.559

https://www.ncbi.nlm.nih.gov/pmc/articles/PMC3746228/

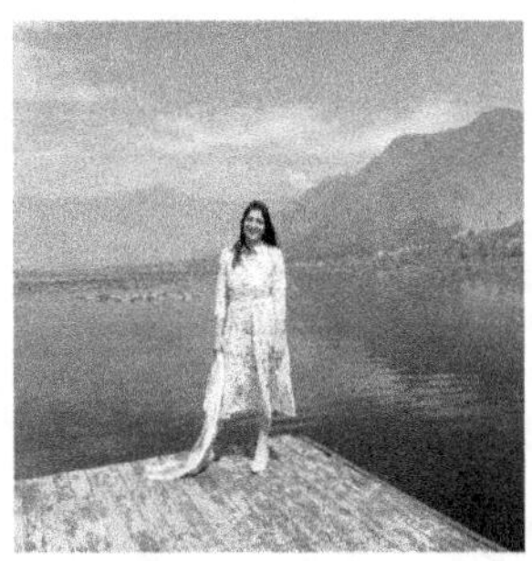

About the Author

author; is on a mission to simplify the journey to holistic well-being. With a personal triumph over the same and blend of expertise I want to inspire positive change. Join me on a wellness adventure through accessible wisdom and transformative insights.